Permanent Hair Removal Solution

A book with Natural remedies to get rid of Facial Hair
Permanently

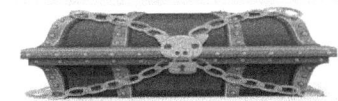

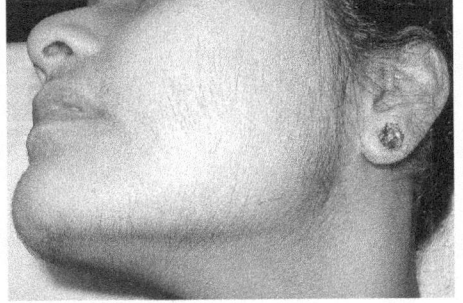

Disclaimer

The information in this eBook reflects the opinions of the author and is not intended to replace medical or psychological advice, or any other professional advice. This EBook is not intended to diagnose or treat any psychological or medical conditions or disorders. If you are in need psychological or medical treatment, consult with a certified and licensed professional before determining whether the information in this book should be used.

© 2015

All rights reserved. No part of this publication may be reproduced, stored in any retrieval system, transmitted, in any form or by any means, electronic, mechanical, photocopying, recording, or otherwise, without prior written consent of the author.

Unwanted Facial Hair

All women have facial and body hair, but the hair is usually very fine and light in color

Excessive or unwanted hair that grows on a woman's face, arms, back, or chest is usually coarse and dark. Women with this condition have characteristics that are commonly associated with male hormones.

Facial hair is normal for both men and women. Hair growth can occur due to hormonal changes. It may be caused by genetics. Unwanted Facial or Body hair/ Excessive Have Growth in Women is also called Hirsutism.

The major reason for Excess Facial Hair is imbalanced Harmones or Excess of Male hormones.

Remedy for Permanent Hair Removal

1. Prosopis cineraria / Sami Seeds

Commonly used Names : Sami, Jand, Jandi, Ghaff

Other Names - Sangri, Khejri.

Procedure : Take the fruits of Prosopis cineraria, Now grind the fruits of Prosopis cineraria and make a paste.

Now first shave the area cleanly where unwanted hair need to be removed.

Apply this paste on the shaved area. Repeat this process for about 3 or 7 times.

After this, the hair will not grow further more and the hair will permanently disappear. Paste of Shami seeds prevents the growth of arm.

Other names of this **Prosopis cineraria** Tree/Plant :
- Jammi chettu (in Telugu)
- Botanical name: Prosopis cineraria
- Other Names
- Arabic (ghaf)
- Bengali (shami)
- Gujarati (khijado,sumri,semru,sami,kamra)
- Hindi (janti,banni,jand,chonksa,sangri,shami,chaunkra,khejiri);
- Sanskrit (jhind,jhand)
- Urdu (jandi,thand,kandi)
- Tamil (perumbay,vanni,jambu)
- General name (jand,kandi,khejri)

Prosopis cineraria occurs in Oman, Saudi Arabia, the United Arab Emirates, Afghanistan, southern Iran, Afghanistan, Pakistan, and India.

In India - Punjab, Western Rajasthan and Gujarat and is common in Bundelkhand and the neighborhoods of Delhi and Agra. It is also found in the dry parts of Central and Southern India, parts of Maharashtra (near Nasik), Andhra Pradesh, Karnataka south of Godavari, Haryana, Western Uttar Pradesh and the drier parts of the Deccan Plateau, Tuticorin.

Below is the picture of **Prosopis cineraria**

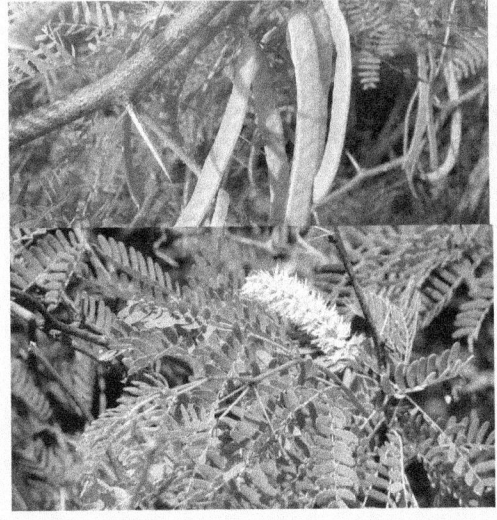

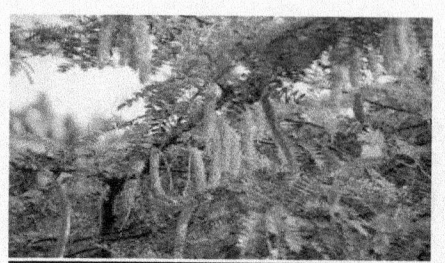

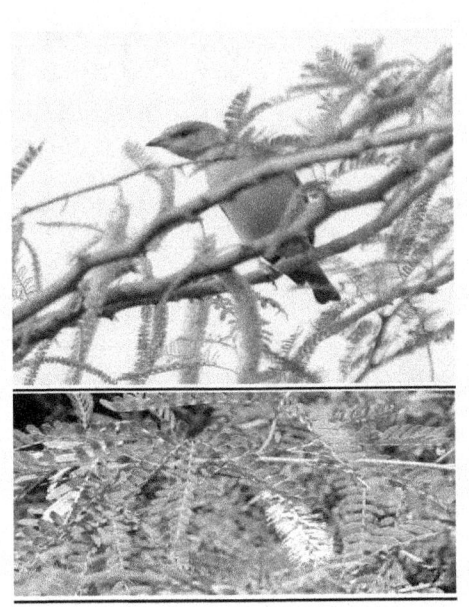

Following are some other methods of hair removal at home but may not permanently remove the hair or may not work on all skin types.

2. Multani Mitti Face Pack

Procedure: Take 3 tablespoon of multani mitti powder. Add a little bit of turmeric and add water or gulabjal according to your need, take that much that it can turn in smooth paste. Apply this paste on your face for 15 minutes. When it gets dry removes it with little water on direction opposite to your hair growth. Do this until your hair start disappearing. If there is excess hair in your face it take some time but don't worry you will get rid of this facial hair.

3. Oatmeal and Banana Face Pack

Procedure: Mix two tablespoons of oatmeal with a ripe banana, and apply this paste on the affected areas. Massage it for 15 minutes, and wash it off with cool water.

This paste will also provide a glowing skin.

4. Potato and Lentil Face Pack

Procedure: Mix a tablespoon of honey, lemon juice each with five tablespoons of potato juice. Grind the lentils (soaked overnight) to a smooth paste. Add all the ingredients and apply the mixture for about 20 minutes on the affected area. Wash it off once it is completely dry.

5. Egg White & Cornstarch Face Pack

Procedure: Mix a tablespoon each of cornstarch and sugar with egg white. Apply this mixture on the areas where you have unwanted hair and peel it off once it is dry.

6. Turmeric Powder & Milk Face Pack

Procedure: Mix turmeric powder with milk and apply on the face. Scrub it off slowly moving your fingers in circular motion, and then wash with cold water.

7. Besan Powder Face Pack

Procedure: Take besan powder in a bowl with little(1/2 tea spoon) oil and milk.
Mix this well to make a smooth and tight paste.
Apply this to your face, and leave it to dry completely.
Now apply little oil to your hands and rub your face, in the upside strokes.
Do this until the besan is completely removed from your face.

8. Turmeric with Honey Face Pack

Procedure: Take 1-tablespoon turmeric powder in a bowl and mix honey to this. Apply this to your face and leave it to dry for 15 minutes and wash it off.

9. Rice Powder & Besan Face Pack

Procedure: Take rice powder of about one Tablespoon ,
Add half table spoon besan powder to this.
add buttermilk ,When the paste turns to a medium consistency,
the take this mixture and apply to your face.
Rub this mixture on your face in the upside strokes for about 15 minutes.Wash this off with cold water.
This is to be done daily for about 15 days for best results.

10. Face pack of Sugar and Lemon Juice

Procedure: Mix two tablespoons of sugar and lemon juice, along with 8-9 tablespoons of water. Heat this mixture until bubbles start to appear and then, let it cool.

Apply it on the affected areas and keep it for about 20-25 minutes. Wash with cold water, rubbing in circular motion.

11. Alum

Procedure: Alum is commonly known as fitkari. Take a tablespoon of alum powder Add rose water to form a thick paste and apply as a face pack. Apply this pack as a thin coat all over the face, wait for it to dry and gently rub in a circular motion and remove the pack.

12.Oatmeal And Honey Face pack

Procedure: Mix 1 tablespoon of oatmeal with 1 tablespoon of honey to make a grainy paste. Apply this mixture to your face and let it set in for 15-20 minutes before rubbing it off with your hands in light circular motion. Wash off with water and pat dry. Start with using this pack daily; slowly reduce to 3-4 times a week.

13. Apricot And Honey Face pack

Procedure: Mix half a cup of apricot and mix it with 2 tablespoons of honey to make a grainy mixture. Apply it on your face, leave for 10 minutes. Now start scrubbing it off from your face with fingertips, in a round circular motion. Continue this for another 5-10 minutes and finally wash off with cold water and welcome to gorgeous skin. Start with 5 times a week and reduce as you go.

14. Papaya And Milk Face pack

Procedure: Mix two cubes of grated green papaya (not ripe) with 1 tablespoon of milk. Make a smooth paste and apply to your face. Leave the pack on for 30 minutes, rub off with moist fingers and then wash off with water. Repeat the process 4-5 times a week for quick results.

15. Face pack of Lemon and Honey

Procedure: Mixing two tablespoons of sugar and lemon juice, and one tablespoon of honey. Heat the mixture for about three minutes and add water to make the mixture thinner, if required.

Once the paste cools down, apply cornstarch on the affected areas and spread the paste in the direction of hair growth. Next, use a wax strip or a cotton cloth, and pull the hair out in the opposite direction of growth.

Important Instructions:

We recommend to try **Prosopis cineraria / Sami Seeds** (remedy no.1 in this book) and see the results.

It is a tested solution for Permanent unwanted hair removal.

Feel free to Try any/all of the methods and check which is suitable for you as all the skin types are different.

For all the Face packs : Initially start with small skin area to check if the face pack suits your skin. If it Suits to your skin then only continue the usage as per instructions.

As all the skin types vary, so we do not guarantee any of treatment mentioned in this eBook.

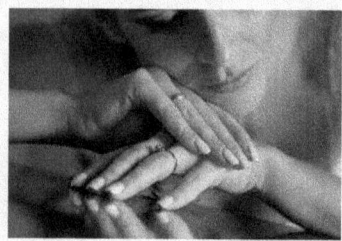

Thank you!

www.ingramcontent.com/pod-product-compliance
Lightning Source LLC
Chambersburg PA
CBHW070915220526
45466CB00005B/2227